YOUR KNOWLEDGE HAS VALUE

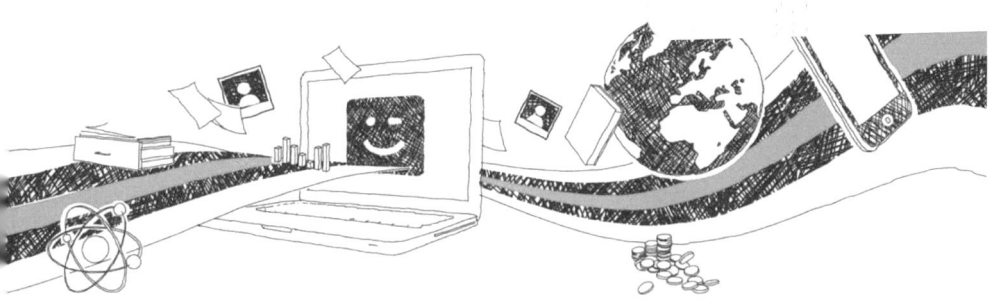

- We will publish your bachelor's and master's thesis, essays and papers

- Your own eBook and book - sold worldwide in all relevant shops

- Earn money with each sale

Upload your text at www.GRIN.com
and publish for free

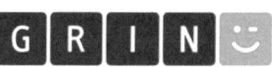

Bibliographic information published by the German National Library:

The German National Library lists this publication in the National Bibliography; detailed bibliographic data are available on the Internet at http://dnb.dnb.de .

This book is copyright material and must not be copied, reproduced, transferred, distributed, leased, licensed or publicly performed or used in any way except as specifically permitted in writing by the publishers, as allowed under the terms and conditions under which it was purchased or as strictly permitted by applicable copyright law. Any unauthorized distribution or use of this text may be a direct infringement of the author s and publisher s rights and those responsible may be liable in law accordingly.

Imprint:

Copyright © 2017 GRIN Verlag
Print and binding: Books on Demand GmbH, Norderstedt Germany
ISBN: 9783668631953

This book at GRIN:

https://www.grin.com/document/411985

Patrick Kimuyu

The Euthanasia Debate

Major Arguments and Religious Perspectives

GRIN Verlag

GRIN - Your knowledge has value

Since its foundation in 1998, GRIN has specialized in publishing academic texts by students, college teachers and other academics as e-book and printed book. The website www.grin.com is an ideal platform for presenting term papers, final papers, scientific essays, dissertations and specialist books.

Visit us on the internet:

http://www.grin.com/

http://www.facebook.com/grincom

http://www.twitter.com/grin_com

Euthanasia Debate

Name: Patrick Kimuyu

Introduction 2
Euthanasia Ethics 2
Major Arguments 3
Religious Perspectives on Euthanasia 4
Conclusion 5
References 6

Introduction

Euthanasia refers to the termination of a terminally ill patient's life (Nicholson, 2000). It is executed at an individual's consent especially when someone is suffering from an incurable health condition. In addition, the decision to terminate a patient's life can also be made by the patient's relatives, the court of law or medical practitioners. However, it is worth noting that the decision by the relatives, the court or the medics is only reached at if the patient is critically ill, such that he or she cannot think or reason. Euthanasia is commonly known as mercy killing or assisted suicide because all the suicide procedures are designed in such a way that, the patient's dignity is not degraded or compromised. The Greeks termed it as *euthanatos* which simply meant easy death (Shiflett & Carroll, 2002). Some individuals who are not terminally ill can sign consent for their lives to be terminated through euthanasia because of ethical reasons especially with matters related to human dignity, but this happens on rare occasions. However, euthanasia has aroused unprecedented debate in the society because it involves several considerations; the most significant one's being practical, religious and ethical issues. Moreover, this practice seems to be somehow challenging to the health professionals, since it is not in alignment with the medical ethics nor legal framework. Euthanasia is illegal in the United Kingdom: thus, it is considered illegal. Therefore, approaches towards euthanasia require caution, since it can lead to legal repercussions (Nicholson, 2000). For instance, voluntary euthanasia is considered as a crime in the United Kingdom, which is punishable by law. Any individual who deliberately executes euthanasia is subjected to serve a jail term. Therefore, this research paper will critically analyze the ethical aspects of euthanasia. Euthanasia is seemingly raising numerous agonizing ethical dilemmas.

Euthanasia Ethics

Euthanasia practice has raised the concern of the society probably because it deals with life. The current debate over euthanasia is seemingly becoming ambiguous because different groups of individuals view it from diverse perspectives. Some individuals consider it to be necessary to terminate the life of a terminally ill patient, who is suffering from an incurable health condition to relieve him or her from pain and suffering. However, it appears somehow difficult to single out the moral differences between euthanasia and normal death because; whether the patient is assisted to die or allowed to get to the eventual normal death, the ultimate result is death (Nicholson, 2000). The second moral dilemma that has made euthanasia appear to confuse is the circumstances under which it is suppose to be executed, since there is a total absence of a consensus justification of euthanasia.

Ordinarily, human beings associate life and death with extremely sensitive ethical values and meaning. They hold the notion that life and death are critical aspects of humanity; therefore, they are solely responsible for making decisions regarding these aspects (Shiflett & Carroll, 2002). In contrast, euthanasia seems to be independently related to the fundamental tenets of humanity, leading to the unprecedented debate in the society.

Major Arguments

In general, arguments over euthanasia are primarily based on practical, religious and ethical issues. The key factors that compel an individual to seek for euthanasia are pain and psychological factors such as depression. Pain caused by disease conditions becomes relatively unbearable at some disease levels. For instance, patients who experience intense pain and suffering because of some health conditions such as breathlessness, incontinence and paralysis consider an early death than prolonged agony caused by pain and discomfort. Recent survey reports that were conducted in the U.S showed that most patients who request for euthanasia face severe physical conditions, which seem to degrade the quality of life. Further survey results showed that a third of patients in the Netherlands seek for euthanasia because of severe pain that is caused by their illnesses (Nicholson, 2000).

Libertarians have become extremely vocal on the euthanasia debate, and their arguments are based primarily on human rights and practical aspects. They argue that dying is a human right and exceptionally personal. Therefore, the decision to choose whether to die or live lies on the individual. They claim that euthanasia is necessary for someone who considers dying, rather than, experiencing unbearable pain, if it does not cause harm to other people. They vehemently insist that an individual's decision on life do not need to be interfered with, since other people do not rightfully decide over one's life. Secondly, libertarians argue that euthanasia can be regulated through defining circumstances at which it can be sought for, in the event that an individual faces severe health conditions (Nicholson, 2000). In addition, they suggest that legitimizing euthanasia will help to reduce the burden on healthcare resources, which are currently strained by high costs of maintaining the terminally ill patients. Therefore, they consider it to be realistic if euthanasia is allowed because it can ensure equitable distribution of healthcare resources.

Moreover, philosophers have posed a utilitarian argument that universality on moral rules can be enhanced through euthanasia. If euthanasia can be universalized, then death can become an option in ones' life: thus, enabling patients who prefer dying than living to receive social justice (Nicholson, 2000). They claim that euthanasia is morally acceptable because it is usually done with the consent of the ailing individual, and it does not infringe upon the rights of other people.

Opponents of euthanasia debate have voiced their concerns too. However, their arguments are extremely diverse because they are based on a number of aspects. These aspects include moral concerns, medical ethics and religious issues.

They argue that euthanasia devalues life because it interferes with the fundamental processes of human life. They claim that death should be perceived as a natural phenomenon like birth and life as a whole (Shiflett & Carroll, 2002). Secondly, opponents of the euthanasia practice argue that it goes against the best interests of the society since individuals hold some degree of value and meaning in the society. Therefore, allowing euthanasia appears to impart elements of fear into someone's life. Thirdly, opponents of euthanasia have raised fears over the regulation of the issue, since it may compromise medical ethics (Nicholson, 2000). For instance, approval of euthanasia as part of the medical procedures may compromise the performance of healthcare professionals (Dobson & Galbraith, 2000). Fourthly, they argue that promoting universality of euthanasia may introduce pressure and abuse. It is feared that some individuals may pressurize terminally ill patients to seek for euthanasia unwillingly (Dobson & Galbraith, 2000). Moreover, antagonists to this debate fear that medics may go against the will of the patients in executing euthanasia, since regulations may give them overall mandate of making vital decisions over the lives of patients.

Religious Perspectives on Euthanasia

From a religious perspective, euthanasia is viewed to as unethical practice because it seems to compromise religious doctrines especially those which are concerned with life and death.

Christians hold that birth and death constitutes the fundamental life processes that were created by God, and they are ought to be respected because they are sacred. They further claim that life is a sacred gift from God which has to be treated with dignity (Shiflett & Carroll, 2002). Muslims claim that life is a sacred gift from Allah and; therefore, human beings do not have any right to decide over birth and death. As such, assisted suicide appears to fall out of the Islamic doctrines. Moreover, Hindus view euthanasia as social vice that may compromise the Karma of patients and medics. In general, the world's popular religions are against euthanasia because it contravenes the fundamental religious doctrines.

Conclusion

In a brief conclusion, euthanasia seems to have raised ethical concerns in the society. Some of the key issues include ethical, practical and religious issues. However, euthanasia encompasses immense ambiguity because there is a total absence of homogeneity in the societal perception. Therefore, different groups of individuals in the society view at the issue from diverse perspectives: thus, leading to the emergence of two opposing sides: the proponents and the opponents.

Proponents of the euthanasia debate argue that it is acceptable, as long as one's decision will not cause harm to the rights of others. In addition, they claim that universality of euthanasia will reduce the burden on healthcare resources. In contrast, opponents of euthanasia maintain that it is unethical in virtually all aspects of human life. They hold a popular notion that death is a natural phenomenon and: therefore, human beings lack the right to interfere with life processes. However, there is no universal consensus over whether euthanasia is right or wrong, leading to the current unprecedented ethical dilemma.

References

Dobson, K., & Galbraith, K. (2000). The Role of the Psychologist in Determining Competence for Assisted Suicide/euthanasia in the Terminally Ill. *Canadian Psychology, 41*, 7-23.

Nicholson, R. (2000). No Painless Death yet for European Euthanasia Debate. *The Hastings Center Report, 30*, 3-16.

Shiflett, D., & Carroll, V. (2002). *Christianity on Trial: Arguments against Anti-Religious Bigotry*. San Francisco, CA: Encounter Books.

YOUR KNOWLEDGE HAS VALUE

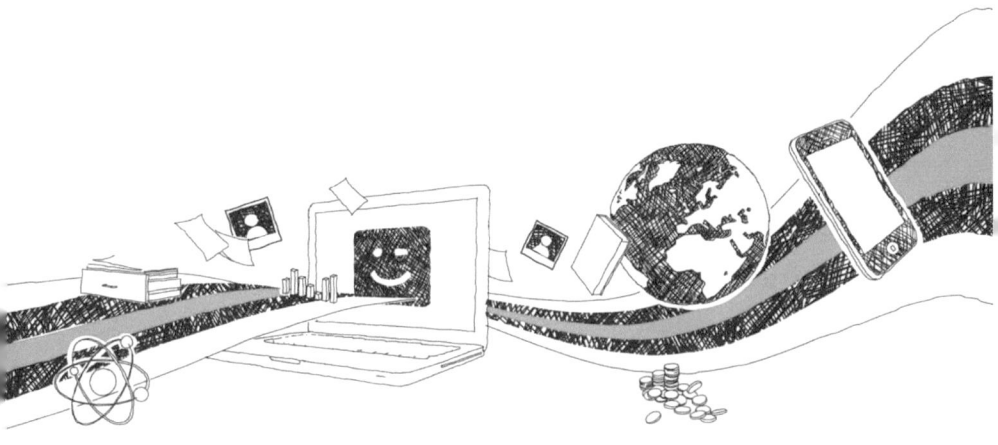

- We will publish your bachelor's and master's thesis, essays and papers

- Your own eBook and book - sold worldwide in all relevant shops

- Earn money with each sale

Upload your text at www.GRIN.com
and publish for free

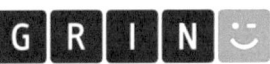